Bernhard J. Schmidt

Plaintext compact

Autism

Flight or Fight

New Perspectives on
Challenging Behaviors

Bernhard J. Schmidt

Plaintext compact
Autism - Flight or Fight
New Perspectives on
Challenging Behaviors

ISBN: 978-3750417922

translated from
Klartext kompakt
Autismus - Flucht oder Kampf
Neue Perspektiven auf herausforderndes Verhalten
© 2018 Bernhard J. Schmidt
ISBN: 978-3748108382

Production and Publishing:
BoD – Books on Demand, Norderstedt, Germany

Bibliographic information of the German National Library:
The German National Library lists this publication
in the German National Bibliography; detailed bibliographic
Data are available online at http://dnb.dnb.de.

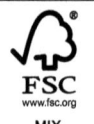

Table of content

I. PREFACE

Like the previous books, this book also leaves the hitherto purely descriptive, that is, phenomenological-descriptive viewpoint. This has not come in the last 50 years, much beyond the descriptions of Hans Asperger and Leo Kanner. These two pioneers are still widely quoted and it is attempted, building on this - all merits - antiquated perspectives not only to understand autistic and challenging behavior of autistics, but also to point out possible intervention.

The following remarks, on the other hand, are based on a uniform social-psychological and development-dynamic theory, which has already been extensively described elsewhere [Schmidt, B.J. 2015/1, 2015/2 ...].

This very first autism theory sheds new light not only on the challenging behavior of autistic individuals, but also on autism and the possibilities of intervention as a whole. Autism is no longer misunderstood as a disease but, on the contrary, as a vulnerability that, in a socio-cultural environment, can lead to disturbances of social interaction and, as a result, disruption of development. Also, the new theory reveals a branch of autism hidden from a phenomenological-descriptive view confined to "shell and hedgehog children" - the "fight" type. These children respond to anxiety and stress as a basic problem of autistics not with "flight" in retreat, rituals and stereotypes, but with "struggle", for example, with pronounced exploration behavior.

In addition to the new theory, the following comments are based above all on the experience of more than 50 families with autistic children in the "Solidar Hotel Goldener Stern". In this a 7-day holiday for families with (autistic) children was offered. In the "Stern" we experienced the autistic children and adolescents with their parents and siblings for a week - in the company and in comparison with other children and their families. Guests were both early childhood, partly mutistic children, who are unfortunately overlooked too often today due to the strong public presence of adult Asperger autistic, to Asperger and highly functional autists of all ages. By relaxing together with other children in a stress-free and safe-feeling environment, it is often not possible for the other guests to distinguish the autistic children from the neurotypical after just a few days.

Probably the nicest compliment in just over a year Solidar Hotel was the following:

An autistic boy came to us and said we probably had a good spell on the Golden Star.

For here he could play with other children together with his Lego, which he otherwise hardly succeeds.

And he wanted to know how to do such a magic ...

My special thanks go therefore to the families with autistic children, who were our guests, and thus have made possible only the following insights.

II. INTRODUCTION

The essential novelty of understanding autism is that a "disruption of SOCIAL INTERACTION" can not be understood solely through the study of autistic individuals. So that one should not only look for the causes and solutions in these alone. And that even autistics, like all humans, can develop on the one hand and on the other need social interaction for their development.

Even the name "autism" and the associated idea that autistics are self-sufficient, is therefore misleading.

The key to developing many, indeed almost all, human capacities lies in social interaction, that is, in interaction with other people.

And the problems for autistics arise because they are not adequately affected by social interaction, e.g. participate in the form of group activities. Either through withdrawal by the autistic individual, isolation by well-intentioned parents, or else through exclusion, bullying and marginalization.

Successful participation in the social interaction of groups is the key to the positive development of autistic individuals.

1   Behavior

Humans "behave" in a physical and social environment. Above all, behavior serves one's own survival and reproduction.

There are innate parts of behaviors, such as exploration and aggression (which I will come back to later). The manifestation of these behaviors is, however, regulated by the participation in the physical and social world, so adapted, and learned.

In the physical environment, ie the world of sensory impressions such as seeing, hearing, smelling, ..., "sensory integration" is learned. So the understanding and the classification of noises, smells ... Through the sensory integration the sensory impressions become understandable and processable.

They no longer appear disordered and incomprehensible and therefore no longer trigger anxiety and stress.

In the social world, on the other hand, and to a large extent unconsciously, almost everything necessary for living together within a group is learned. Be it the evaluation of events (event appraisal), which emotions fit to which event and in which intensity these emotions are shown [Smith, Bond (1998)], rules of social interaction, emotion regulation, language, ...

Social interaction is learned by people through social interaction!

So if a person is separated from participation in social interaction, whether through withdrawal or exclusion, it leads to a disruption of these learning processes - and then often to challenging behavior.

2   Challenging behavior

Which behaviors are so far attributed to the challenging behavior, and thus interpreted as such?

„*"Challenging behavior" includes behaviors*
• with self-hazard
- extroverted, so visible to the outside as to run away, beating, scratching, biting, mutilating, swallowing things
- introverted, that is to say inward like social indifference, not talking, withdrawal through self-stimulation, disruption of the day / night rhythm

• with foreign hazard
- threaten, spit, bite, scratch, beat, force someone to sex, etc.
• which are perceived as disturbing in cohabitation
- excrement, frequent vomiting, screaming, stereotypical

handling of objects, tics, vocalizations, rigid insistence on routine, unruly behavior, entering unfamiliar spaces, keeping no distance, etc.
• which are experienced as psychologically conditioned
- anxiety, depression, hyperactivity, autism or psychosis, but also self- and auto-aggression, etc.
• associated with property damage and / or abnormal handling of property
- destroying own or foreign property, pyromania, etc.
- Compulsive handling of objects, stealing, hiding or swallowing things "
[from: Wege zur Teilhabe – Herausforderndes Verhalten von Menschen mit Behinderungen. Handreichung des Lebenshilfe-Landesverbandes Bayern 2017]

Autism as such and its attendant behaviors are perceived as challenging behaviors per se - and are diagnosed as virtually inevitable and uncontrollable by a diagnosis.
That's wrong!
In a later chapter, the cited enumeration will be corrected under the new perspective.

3 „Problems" with challenging behavior

The demarcation and understanding of challenging behavior are in principle, not only in the area of autism, accompanied by a number of problems.

3.1 It can be part of an adequate but also of a disturbed development.

Even though this can or should hardly be perceived in a soft-flushed affluent society, aggression and exploration are firmly anchored in the behavioral repertoire not only of humans but of mammals and other living beings as well.

Exploration and aggression serve to explore and defend territory, food, sexual partners ... At the same time they also serve to explore social structures and boundaries as well as their position within the group.

Conflict and confrontation are therefore a fixed and necessary component of social interaction!

Challenging behavior can thus be a normal and necessary part of an adequate development and can occur again and again in defiant and mob phases not only during adolescence.

If this behavior, which is part of a normal development, is falsely labeled as challenging, then it can lead to challenging behavior as a "self-fullfilling prophecy"!

On the other hand, challenging behavior can also be an expression of a disturbed development, in which e.g. the sensory integration, emotion regulation ... were not sufficiently learned.

3.2   It can have psychological as well as physical and social causes.

The causes for challenging behavior can be manifold. In order to provide at least a little clarity, a distinction is made between physical, social as well as psychological causes.

3.2.a   Physical

Due to the often associated with autism hypersensitivity and stimulation filter weakness, it can come to a meltdown, so a failure of all regulatory mechanisms, for example, due to a sensory overload. With the result of uncontrolled behavior like hitting, biting, spitting ....
But also "sensory integration" can and must be learned by

participation in physical and social life. Also by autistic people!

The shielding of autists from the environment is well meant, but ultimately counterproductive. On the other hand, it makes sense to keep dealing with the environment in the area of stress balance. [Schmidt, B.J.; Ganz, A. (2016)]

3.2.b   Social

In the area of social causes, on the other hand, a distinction must be made between passive and active. In the case of passive causes, the autistic individual does not understand the social environment in its often irrational and group-dependent behavior. This can lead to anxiety and stress and, as a consequence, challenging behavior. And in the form of "flight" by retreating into stereotypes and rituals, auto-aggression ...

But also by "fight" in the form of strong exploration, to investigate the environment for possible dangers, as well as aggression against other ...

It is far too short to look for the causes of challenging behavior, especially in autistic people, only in the physical environment or in the autistic person himself. NT people (neurotypical people - without autism) unconsciously expect participation in each group in the form of conformity, imitation of behaviors and fashions, small-talk ...

People who do not show these behaviors are excluded from participation. And the constant exclusion from group communication is already bullying! [Schmidt, B.J. (2016)]

So also groups can, for example in the form of mobbing, show socially inadequate behavior. As a result, the victims of bullying often show challenging behavior. Or the victim's behavior is defined as challenging to justify the group's bullying behavior. [Schmidt, B.J. (2016)]

Bullying against clients can also occur in teachers, therapists, educators and nurses!

So if autistic people run amok, then - as a rule - profound bullying experiences are the cause, and not autism as such!

3.2.c   Psychological

All people, whether "normal", mentally disabled or autistic, can develop mental disorders. As a result of this disorder again challenging behavior can occur. In the field of autism, anxiety disorders (for example, social phobia), obsessive-compulsive disorders, but also dissociative personality disorders should be mentioned here [Schmidt, B.J.; Ganz, A. (2016)]. Although a differential diagnosis is difficult, especially in the field of mental disability, this should not be ruled out. Again, a frivolous labeling and attribution that the cause of the challenging behavior lies solely in the mental disability or autism, can be very hindering.

3.3   Behavior is subject to interpretation

Challenging behavior occurs within and is defined by the cultural-historical social environment. What is considered challenging in one culture may be considered normal in another culture.
If, for example, it is expected in our culture to look into the eye, to show hand and feelings, the opposite is true in Japan.
The interpretation of the behavior of a person also depends heavily on the affiliation to the respective group. The same act, which is considered "cool" for accepted group members, can be seen as a challenge by outsiders [Schmidt, B.J., Döhler C. u. D. (2018)].

3.4   Different perspectives

What is interpreted as "challenging" from the perspective of the group often makes sense from the perspective of the autistic, though not always purposeful.

It is a fundamental mistake of many so-called "therapies" of the last decades to try to decrease through training those behaviors that are necessary and meaningful from an autistic perspective.

However, stimming, rituals and stereotypical behaviors, as well as exploration and aggression often have their causes in anxiety and stress, and serve to reduce them.

In a technologically prosperous society, the physical environment as well as the behavior of NT people is a permanent challenge from an autistic point of view!

First, because of the, often associated with autism, hypersensitivity and irritant filter weakness.

Second, because NT people are not as conscious, rational and autonomous as they like to believe. To a large extent, NT people are unconscious, irrational and group-dependent. We will come back to it.

3.5 Different characteristics

Another difficulty in identifying challenging behavior and planning an intervention is that even in one and the same person can

- lead a cause (physical, mental or social) to various challenging behaviors and

- the same challenging behavior have different causes.

Practical example: Luis, 7 years old, early childhood, hardly speaking autistic:

Luis had "discovered" the throwing of objects for himself. He showed this in almost all possible causes, which are explained below.
Once it was simply an impulse and lacked the necessary impulse control.
Then again, there was a lack of frustration tolerance, the cause of throwing, e.g. with the salt shaker.
But even if the mother talked to me, for example, and he did not have the full attention, he threw things around. Because he had learned that he always receives full attention in case of misconduct.

But sometimes it was simply mobbing to test the limits of his actions.

III. AUTISM

Imagine, an anthropologist (human explorer) from Mars lands by accident in a surgical department of a hospital. So he gets the impression that all people have a bandage or plaster at any point.

People without dressing and plaster are not recognized as such by this Martian.

Autism research faces the same problem. Autism was first observed in children who had some disorders due to various factors to be described.

Thus, autism has been and still is considered a disease. Autists who have not developed disorders were and are not perceived as such.

The definition of autism does not go beyond the limit of a diagnosis, which presupposes a disturbance, ultimately in the form of challenging behavior.

Autism is NOT a disease, NO disorder, and NO disability.
Autism is a vulnerability within a culture-historical environment.

On the one hand, there are adults who live normally and integrated into society, without diagnosis, without challenging behavior, and who are nevertheless autistic. On the other hand, at the Solidar Hotel, we have children who have all the typical characteristics of autistic people, such as show in the game behavior, but are normally developed. Again, there would be no diagnosis, because neither a suffering nor a developmental disorder would be noted.

Added to this were historical processes that have led to a static view of autism in research and general understanding [Schmidt, B.J. (2019/1)]. Over the past 50 years, autistic individuals have been denied the opportunity to develop and discredited development-dynamic approaches.
But also autistic children can develop.

Accompanying this was necessarily the misconception that autistics are themselves enough, can not and do not want to communicate. And so the dogma that autistic people can not develop and therefore do not need any social interaction was born. This dogma still works today - with fatal consequences for autistic people.
However, autistic children also need social interaction for both their development and mental health.

In the case of autistic children, only the deficits were considered through the above points, focusing only on the deviations as well as challenging behavior. All behavior was understood as a solid, unchanging part of autism. **But autistic children are above all children with the normal behavior of children. With anger, fear and defiance, exploration behavior including the attempt to test limits ...**

1   But what is autism?

If you say goodbye to the mistakes of the past 50 years
and consult the findings of social psychology, then it
quickly becomes clear and explainable what autism is.
For a long time it has been described that autistic people
hardly show facial expressions and gestures and do not
imitate their counterparts, are having a hard time with
small-talk ... these are the innate, largely inherited and
autistic characteristics!

Social psychology shows that precisely these behaviors,
which do not show autistics, serve the unconscious (!)
group communication.
People are only too happy to perceive themselves as
individuals who act independently, consciously and
rationally.
However, the results of social psychology in recent years
and decades paint a different picture.
People unconsciously orient themselves towards the
behavior of the respective group and imitate it. This
imitation extends all the way to motor processes. Autists
often have difficulties with the motor skills or the
movements look strange, since they do not imitate the
behavior of the other people.

The behavior of NT people is so much less conscious and rational than people like to think.

It is much more unconscious and therefore often irrational group behavior.

Orientation to the group through unconscious group communication serves NT people (neurotypical people - that is, without autism) as an "autopilot".

The unconscious group communication takes place via exactly the behaviors that autistics do not show. Namely about facial expressions, gestures, imitation, modulation of voice, synchronization ... as well as small-talk.

Autistic people therefore lack the unconscious group communication and thus the unconscious orientation on the group, ie the "autopilot". This means that autistics always have to orient themselves and decide. Autists have to build their own perception and decision-making structures.

This is why autistic people are literally in the truest sense of the word and in no way pejoratively "behaviorally original", the heterogeneity of autistic people ("If you know an autistic person ... you know exactly one autistic person") will find its explanation here.

On the other hand, the active orientation and the large number of decisions to be made costs a lot of time and energy.

Opportunities for retreat and rest are essential for the healthy development of autistic individuals.

More importantly, NT people need unconscious group behavior as a kind of social "grooming" and thus expect the opposite. As a rule, autistic individuals are noticeable because they do not show this behavior.

But even though autistic children lack "**unconscious** group communication and interaction," this does not mean that they are not capable of "**social** communication and interaction." It does not mean that they do not need them for their development - on the contrary.

"But inclusion is not simply a passive tolerating of the presence of a physically or mentally different individual, but an active and continuous process.
Inclusion is not simply being allowed to "be there", but always is an invitation, request and encouragement to participate in social interaction." [Schmidt 2016]

Promoting the development of autistic individuals, whether children, adolescents or adults, always requires a successful social interaction.

2   Anxiety and Stress

Anxiety and stress are the main problems and antagonists for autistic development. Because anxiety and stress prevent social interaction [Dykema, Ravi (2006)]. Safety and relaxation are therefore the prerequisites for social interaction, because fear and stress put people in a "flight or fight" mode, which is characterized by high concentrations of the stress hormones adrenaline and cortisol. The often-encountered physical and mental health problems of autistic people are often due to a permanent state of stress [Schmidt, B.J.; Ganz, A ., (2016)].
But how come the particular susceptibility of autistic people to anxiety and stress?

2.1   Hypersensitivity and filter weakness

For many autistic people, as already mentioned, there is a sensory hypersensitivity, which means that autistic people perceive the sensory stimuli of the environment much more intensively. Be it noises, light stimuli ... and above all smells, which can have a very direct influence on our emotions.
At the same time, unlike NT people, the disturbing

29

stimuli are not automatically filtered out, there is a lack of stimulus filter in many autistic.

Whether the ticking of a clock, the cries of other children in the day care center, the smell of the cleaning agent, the flickering of the neon tube, the much too bright light ... everything patters unfiltered on the autistic child and thereby generates in this stress.

But hypersensitivity and irritant filter weakness are of course only a possible concomitant of autism. The real core is the lack of the "autopilot" in the form of unconscious group communication.

2.2   Anxiety Avoiding as a group goal

An essential task of groups is the avoidance of anxiety (anxiety avoiding). Shared behavior reduces the fear of each group member. But without unconscious group communication, autistic individuals are often excluded from groups and thus from the possibility of anxiety reduction.

On the other hand, groups often behave irrationally due to the "autopilot", the unconscious group communication. Also, this irrational behavior of groups can cause anxiety and stress in autistic people.

2.3   Consequences of anxiety and stress

The combination of hypersensitivity, irritant filter weakness, and lack of the "autopilot" often results in high anxiety and stress levels in autistic individuals.
As a result, in addition to the health problems already mentioned, the following three behaviors can be observed:

2.3.a   Avoidance of change

The avoidance of change and the insistence on the always same processes or for example ways is a frequently encountered feature in autistic people - but also in groups [Menzies Lyth, I. (1960)]. Only this behavior, ie the avoidance of change, is rarely noticed in groups, because everyone participates. In the end, insisting on known structures and behaviors leads to the elimination of anxiety - whether in groups or autistic individuals.
But the avoidance of change, often mistakenly presented as irrevocably, if not desirably, by adult autists, naturally hinders development. It follows that trying out new ways and behaviors should be practiced - at least initially in the safest possible environment. And only if there is enough energy left in the autistic child.

2.3.b   Insistence on sameness

The insistence on always the same processes, also e.g. while playing, of course, is the flip side of avoiding change. The same rituals and processes are familiar and thus provide security in a world that appears to be insecure and often incomprehensible.

2.3.c   Aggressive behavior

Life means the ongoing struggle against the automatic process of decay while using energy.
To ensure survival, some basic strategies are found on living beings in general.
Above all, it is the search for food (energy) and (sexual) propagation. In order to secure these processes, there are added as "auxiliary services", without claim to completeness:

- Exploration behavior (exploration behavior). The environment is explored time and again to find food sources and sexual partners.

- Aggression - to defend territory, food and sexual partners against competitors, and to defend themselves as well as the brood against predators.

- Stress - as a physiological response to a threat to equip the body for flight or fight.

- Social behavior - to enable (over) life in a group.

All auxiliary services are so first of all "normal" and live useful. Not just social behavior, but also exploration and aggression.

IV. „FIGHT OR FLIGHT" CHILDREN

So far, the importance of anxiety and stress has largely been overlooked in the context of autism.

Behaviors that occur as a result of anxiety and stress have been and are erroneously used as diagnostic criteria.

But it is anxiety and stress that have a significant impact on both the development and behavior of autistic individuals.

Nature offers two types of behavior under fear and stress:

- Flight, or

- Fight

But only the escape behavior in the form of withdrawal and e.g. stereotypical behavior, aggression against oneself (autoaggression) ... was equated with autism (keyword "hedgehog children", "shell children"). Autistic children who do not show this inward escape behavior, but respond to anxiety and stress with "combat", ie with aggression against other, increased exploration behavior, etc., were diagnosed with difficulty as (untypical) autistic individuals. However, at the Solidar Hotel, we experience again and again autistic children of one and the other type. Just the distinction in the "Fight type" and "Flight type" is helpful especially in the context of challenging behavior.

1   Practical examples

Flight-child: Andreas, 6 years, infantile autism and mutistic.
The family of Andreas came with some discomfort to us in the Solidar Hotel Goldener Stern, but had failed the previous holiday attempt. Andreas had screamed at the time of the arrival at the resort in the car and refused to leave the car, that the family was back immediately. That's how the parents wanted to see how long Andreas would endure in the Golden Star.
Andreas was completely withdrawn at the beginning and showed self-destructive behavior (aggression against himself) in the form of a head beat against the wall.
The family stayed with us the whole week and during this time completed an AuJA start week, a child-initiated support program (www.auja.org). Due to the funding program, Andreas's behavior became more relaxed and open day by day. Negative beliefs, which are often found in parents of autistic children, such as "Andreas does not play with the ball", were refuted by him more and more.

Fight-children: Simon, Joshua, Jonas ...

These children are very restless at the beginning, running around the house, exploring every corner, every room, every drawer. As we understand the importance and need for the children, exploration is not only allowed in the Solidar Hotel - we are happy about it. And we see exploration as a valuable way to build social interaction! The kitchen is always a special attraction for children - and they are allowed to enter, play with the dishshower, start the dishwasher ... we explain the many large kitchen appliances. And that too, and especially the children, who at first sight would deny the cognitive abilities necessary for understanding. By being able to check the environment for hazards and perceive it to be safe, the children then relax quite quickly and show amazing positive developments as a result.

1.1   Autism and ADHD

It may be a daring but obvious proposition that autistic people of the "fight" type at least often receive the diagnosis of ADHD. And conversely, people with an ADHD diagnosis are actually autistic "fight" -type. People with an initial ADHD diagnosis often receive an autism diagnosis later in life.

V. CHALLENGING BEHAVIOR AND INTERVENTIONS

An important distinction regarding the understanding of challenging behavior and possible intervention is the already mentioned between "flight" and "fight" type.

1   The „flight"-type

The withdrawal into stereotypes, rituals and self-injurious behavior of autistic people is - pedagogically seen - the biggest challenge!

These autistic people have fled to their inner world from a world perceived as foreign, hostile and threatening.

They build rituals and stereotypes into an understandable and familiar world.

It can be a long way to give children and young people back the necessary trust and access back to the world.

Please refer to the book "Klartext kompakt. Frühkindlicher Autismus. Verstehen = Helfen"[Ganz, A .; Schmidt, B.J. (2016) - Translation in preparation], in which Ganz and I present the child-centered and child-initiated support programs for DIR / Floortime, Son-Rise®, AuJA and Mifne suitable for the "flight" agents.

1.1 Excursus: Limits and dangers of child-initiated support programs

So gut und geeignet die kindzentrierten Förderprogramme für autistische Kinder vom „flight"-Typ sind,
also für Kinder, die einen Kontakt mit der Welt ver-
weigern und sich komplett in ihre eigene Welt zurück
gezogen haben, so haben diese Förderprogramme doch
auch ihre Grenzen und Gefahren.

1.1.a Limits

The playroom in which support program usually takes
place is always an artificial world. And the interaction, as
good as it is to re-establish communication in the
beginning, remains artificial. So, these support programs
are good for getting started with interacting with people.
But social interaction is learned through social interaction
- and that takes place in the real world with all its dangers
and risks, and especially in peer groups.
Once the first stages of interaction within the playroom
have been achieved, further interventions such as social
skills training would be necessary as offers.
And with the "fight" type, which explores the
environment strongly, it does not make much sense to

bring these children back into a playroom. Here, the opportunity should be seized to use exploration to build a relationship.

Likewise, the child-initiated support programs quickly reach their limits in aggressive behavior. Too much effort is made to build up an interaction so that, for fear of a renewed withdrawal of the child, there are hardly any limits to aggressive action.

1.1.b   Dangers

The biggest danger of child-initiated support programs is not to see the limits listed above.

For example, a family with a very aggressive juvenile autistic who had years of "playroom" was advised to use even more Son-rise® to solve the problem. Its own boundaries were ignored and instead followed the principle of "more of the same".

On the other hand, in almost all, not only the child-initiated support and therapy programs but also e.g. at ABA, made the parents "co-therapists". From now on, the behavior of the children will be documented by the parents from a "therapeutic meta-level", analyzed and, if in doubt, discussed with the children ("What does it matter to you if you throw the salt shaker?"). A normal interaction between parents and children, in which there is room for conflict and the child is once even reprimanded, is thereby prevented. But the social interaction with the parents - and that at eye level - is of central importance to development. Even the parents of autistic children should and must remain parents - and not become "experts in their own right".

Another, partly also from financial interests bred error is that of the "much helps much". The support program then determines the entire life of the entire family and is run around the clock as possible. You rush from appointment to appointment, from therapy to therapy.

"We no longer have friends but only people around us who pay for their participation in the therapies. We do not have any time left to go through the many therapies," says a mother. But how is the young autistic son of this mother to learn what friends are and how to deal with them, if the parents themselves have no friends?

2   The „fight"-type

On the other hand, exploratory children of the "fight" type are more strenuous, but also easier to guide, in which the urge to exploration is used and channeled into appropriate channels. To a child showing exploration and aggression, one can show necessary boundaries but also the world and everything that can be discovered in it - a child, on the other hand, who has retreated into his own world, has his own, ultimately hostile to life , Limits set. In any case, the avoidance of unfortunately occurring misinterpretations of the (challenging) behavior is necessary.

3   Misinterpretations

A wrong interpretation of a supposedly challenging behavior necessarily leads astray. Unfortunately, the field of autism research is full of judgmental assumptions and concepts that stand in the way of understanding and thus successful intervention.

3.1   „Running away tendency"

As a rule, the "away" in the "running away tendency" is superfluous in the area of autism and leads to false conclusions.
Autists very often have a very high state of arousal, which can manifest itself in many areas.
For example, through teeth grinding, a posture of arms and hands reminiscent of a spasticity, and also by a "running tendency", which serves to reduce tension. So the goal is not the "away" but the "running". If this is understood correctly, the "problem" can be remedied by

sufficient movement in the form of running and other stress reduction.

If the urge to move is understood as a "running tendency", the reaction, for example, of the parents also changes.

Practical example 1

Due to the changed perception that her 17-year-old son of Asperger did not want to "walk away", but just wanted to walk, and he was also so oriented that he could always find his way back, the parents responded calmly to his son's long trips in the forest landscape of the Fichtelgebirge, where the Solidar Hotel is located.
No further "search actions" were started.

Practical example 2

After pointing out the misinterpretation of the running "away", the parents responded that they would stick to their son running away. Because the 16-year-old son with early childhood autism would always run to playgrounds to take away children there baby dolls, for which he had a special interest. But the problem here was not running "away", but the inadequate goal of taking away the dolls from children.

3.2 Because the child behaves differently, that he has a mental retardation.

People expect, unconsciously, the participation in group behavior among other things by imitation and conformity. The evaluation of an information also depends on the affiliation of the informant to the respective group:

„ The perceived validity of information is always a function of social and relational factors such as the perceived source of a message, the degree to which it has consensual support and the degree to which the target defines the source as a positive reference group, that is, the degree to which it is in line with ingroup norms. So-called informational influence is not purely cognitive but social and normative. There is in fact no way of defining persuasive or valid information independently of the social context within it is apprehended. The same information which persuades one group will fail to persuade another. One group´s expert is another´s crank. One does not accept influence from experts because of the information they provide (if one is not an expert, how can one judge its quality?), but accepts the information as valid because one defines them as an expert (Moscovici, 1976) " [Turner (2005)]

Since autistic children and adolescents generally do not behave in accordance with the group, ie do not show the expected behavior, they are often - and unjustly - alleged to have an intellectual disability.

Practical example: Sebastian, 6 years, „fight-type":
Not only did Sebastian have a diagnosed mental retardation, he also got only negative feedback from the day care center. At the Solidar Hotel he was very active during his first stay at the beginning, explored the whole house and also showed a lot of aggression against his younger sister. His attention span lasted only seconds. However, we could not notice any decrease in intelligence. He was e.g. weasel-quick in the operation of (like foreign) mobile phones. Problems with the German language could be attributed to the bilingualism of the family.
After a few days, Sebastian was much calmer and was able to spend some time, for example, on computational tasks.
On the second visit Sebastian was altogether much calmer, showed hardly any aggression ...
After experiencing how "normal" her child could be with us at the Solidar Hotel, she had successfully intervened at the daycare center on a more neutral view of Sebastian's behavior.

3.3   Explorationis not understood.

It has already been stated that exploration is a normal part of human behavioral patterns. And also the importance for the "fight" children was shown.

If exploration is not understood as necessary for the autistic and is not used to build a relationship, it will cause unnecessary problems.

Practical example:

It sometimes takes a few tries until we can convince the parents of autistic children in the Solidar Hotel that their exploration behavior is not only allowed in our house, but is actually desirable. If initially the autistic children are "captured" by their parents or siblings, the positive use of exploration behavior quickly leads to positive behavioral changes in the autistic children as well as the parents. The children visit us e.g. in the kitchen, but leave them when we ask them. Children, who otherwise hardly get rid of their parents, then move around the house and play with other children.

3.4 Parts of an adequate development are understood as typically autistic.

It has already been mentioned, but one can not say enough that autistics also go through the normal stages of development, albeit perhaps delayed, and thus have defiance and mob phases. If these are dismissed as typically autistic and the limits and rules of social coexistence are not shown, real problems only arise later.

3.5 Parts of an inadequate development are understood as typically autistic.

Because challenging behavior is a basic component of the (until today false) diagnostic criteria, it is quickly said "he's just like that". Thus, it is overlooked that the challenging behavior, however, can only be a symptom of a treatable (in the sense of a pedagogical or psychological intervention) disorder of development.
Also, the autist is thereby deprived of any criticism and correction of his behavior. But especially criticism, but of course praise as well, would be important for both orientation and development.

VI. CAUSES OF CHALLENGING BEHAVIOR

The possibilities for challenging behavior are so varied that it is neither sensible nor possible to enumerate them. It is more important to distinguish the different causes. Because only then can you successfully carry out appropriate interventions.

1   Adequate development

For one thing, challenging behavior can also be part of normal development.
For neurotypical children and adolescents, however, this would not be described as challenging.
Since autistic individuals have so far been denied developmental perspectives and autism has been defined as a disease, it has so far been overlooked that even autistic children and adolescents can follow a normal course of development. In this development, it may then come to normal "challenging" behaviors.

1.1   Mobbing

The "mobbing" should be synonymous here for, as part of a normal development necessary, the exploration of social rules, structures and boundaries. It takes the form of a clear environmental question: "May I do that? How far can I go?"

Intervention
Autistic children and adolescents lack unconscious orientation in different groups - the autopilot is missing. It is therefore to be expected that the "question" about rules and boundaries will be made clearer and more frequent. A central and common mistake is to regard this normal behavior as autistic and ignore it. However, the clear identification of rules and limits as well as the regulation of aggression and exploration are particularly important for autistics.

The faster and clearer the social structure and its boundaries are shown, the better.

For borders not only limit, they also give security and orientation! A child who knows no limits is also completely overwhelmed with his (misunderstood) role as a "boss".

In the Solidar Hotel we see again and again autistic

children and also adolescents, partly also mutistic, who already have the whole family at the age of 5 or 6 years under control. They have their own court, their own entourage. The normal orientation of the children to the parents is reversed - the parents are instead completely oriented to the child.

By tolerating the "normal" taunts, challenging behaviors can then arise due to a disturbed development (e.g., impulse control, frustration tolerance ...).

Due to the lack of autopilot, autistic people especially need clear limits!

2   Disturbed or delayed development

In addition to behaviors that are part of adequate development, autistic individuals have challenging behaviors due to disturbed or delayed development. Important for the understanding and thus an intervention is the clarification of the causes of the challenging behavior. To regard this simply as typical of autism leads astray and can ultimately lead to an amplification of the challenging behavior!

Autistic people with a diagnosis need therapeutic support in any case, as the diagnosis is an expression of a disturbed development. The goal should always be the restoration of a largely normal social interaction as the basis for a normal, especially socio-emotional development.

2.1   Intervention – Fundamentals

If it comes to challenging behavior, then there are two things to consider:
On the one hand, it is primarily anxiety and stress that trigger the challenging behavior.
As the basis of any intervention, the reduction of anxiety and stress is indispensable.
On the other hand, challenging behavior, if not part of an adequate development, is always the result of an already persistent developmental disorder. As in "Autism - Sexuality - Partnership" [Schmidt, B.J .; Döhler, C .; Döhler, D. (2017)] described, an intervention that only wants to eliminate the current problem and ignores the underlying disruption of development is too brief. Therefore one should distinguish in particular with oneself or other endangering behavior between an

1. acute action to prevent this behavior, and
2. an intervention to eliminate possible causes of the disruption of development and to catch up with the affected parts of development.

Of course, keep the child from banging his head on the wall bloody. But this is an acute action to avert the danger, and no intervention in the sense of a pedagogical-psychological measure.

2.2   Attention

As in "Autism and Dog" [Schmidt, B.J. (2019/2)] described, many families focus their activities completely on the autistic child. And on the other to its deficits and negative behaviors. On the other hand, positive behaviors of the autistic child are either barely noticed or not acknowledged to the child by praise as such. But all children need praise, not only for orientation, but also to be perceived as valuable and desired.
The one-sided focus, on the other hand, teaches the autistic child that it is always the center of attention and, secondly, that it gets full attention especially when it proves to be challenging.
In combination with the lack of boundaries because they were not and will not be set, then the development can escalate so that parents consider installing a "time out room" in-house, which is actually a "panic room" because you can no longer cope with the aggression of the growing autistic.

Intervention
Ultimately, a learning process, especially with parents or

caregivers, is necessary to shift the focus and clearly show the rules and limits for social behavior.

During the visits to the dog school of Sylvia Ulrich we were able to achieve good results here, which unfortunately could not always be established by the parents in the long run.

Working with the dogs, on the one hand, distracted the focus from the autistic child and, on the other hand, the parents, by working with the dogs, noticed the importance of praise and reward as a means of orientation.

2.3   Problems with

The variety of difficulties so far presented, such as the lack of autopilot, misinterpretation of behavior e.g. as typical of autism and errors, can then lead to a disturbed socio-emotional development and thus to triggers of challenging behavior.

2.3.a   Impulse control

The autistic has not learned not to put his impulses into action immediately. A common, and often regarded as typically autistic problem. Of course, autistic people can and should also learn how to deal with their own impulses, be they aggressive or not (!).

2.3.b   Frustration tolerance

Essentially, the same thing applies to the lack of frustration tolerance as to impulse control.
The combination of lack of frustration tolerance with lack of impulse control creates an "explosive" mixture.
Frustration tolerance can and should be learned by autistic children and adolescents. But they will not do so if the parents, in anticipatory obedience, fulfill the wishes of the autistic children, which have not yet been expressed.

2.3.c   Emotion regulation

Although impulse control and frustration tolerance are important parts of emotional regulation, it goes beyond that.
On the one hand, the ability to regulate emotions depends heavily on self-esteem and arises through participation in groups [Schmidt, B.J. (2015/2)].
On the other hand, the type and expression of an emotion becomes an event, as already mentioned, in a cultural-historical context, ie also through group participation.

The erroneous "theory" that autistics have no feelings is wrong. Often, only the culture-specific rules for showing one's emotions are not learned.

Interventions

Impulse control, frustration tolerance and also flexibility have to be learned. On the one hand, autistic people should therefore be shown the social limits and rules. Since often only the socio-emotional, but not the cognitive development is affected, this goes beyond a certain age as an appeal to reason.

Practical example: Franz, 12-year-old Asperger

Everything was immediately negatively commented by Franz. The Golden Star would not be a real hotel, the food would not be as expected ... Ultimately a continuing attack on everything and everyone.

Asked about his plans for the future, Franz said that he would start a business with a loan and then get rich. On my then following question, whether he would believe that in his behavior anyone would give a loan, not only thinking, but also learning processes began with him.

On the other hand, social interaction, including participation in different groups, is a necessary prerequisite for learning social interaction! The idea of sending autistic children to online schools is understandable at first glance. But schools are not just a means of imparting knowledge, but are above all places of social interaction!

2.4   In response

It is not enough to point out and raise awareness that autistic people are at great risk of becoming victims of bullying and physical and sexual violence and exploitation. [Schmidt, B.J. (2016)], [Schmidt, B.J .; Döhler, C .; Döhler, D. (2018)].
If autistic has challenging behavior, it should always be considered that this is a response to the above risks.

Interventions
The most important intervention here is the prevention! It should not even come to such acts of violence against autistics. Sensitivity is necessary, but not always easy. Even in care facilities, schools, etc., bullying and violence can also emanate from the supervisors, teachers, etc. The consequences for the victim are usually devastating.

In an acute event this is of course to stop. On the other hand past violent experiences should be worked up psychotherapeutically.

2.5   Overload / Melt down

At the onset of a meltdown, the failure of the regulatory mechanisms with the consequence of, for example, screaming, beating, spitting ... three components are involved.

First, it is the "hard-wired", ie hypersensitivity and stimulus filter weakness.

Secondly, it is the sensory integration that organizes the sensory stimuli through learning processes and thus makes them understandable and trains how to deal with them.

Third, because of the lack of autopilot and irritant filter weakness, autistic individuals need a lot of energy to maintain the necessary regulatory mechanisms.

If either the sensory flood is too strong, the sensory integration was not completed or simply the required energy is missing, it can lead to the collapse of the regulation. Challenging behavior is then a possible consequence.

Interventions

On the one hand, the sensory sensitivity increases together with the stress level. When the body enters fight-or-flight mode, the senses are even more sensitized to detect potential dangers in good time. Therefore, reducing anxiety and stress, as always, is an important part of the intervention.

On the other hand, both the necessary active orientation and the active filtering out of disturbing noises (the automatic stimulus filters are missing or are only weak) consume a lot of energy. If this energy is no longer sufficient, the regulatory mechanisms collapse.

Furthermore, sensory integration is also learned. Providing permanent protection for people with sunglasses and ear protection robs them of the possibility of learning how to deal with even unpleasant stimuli. This learning of sensory integration should, of course, take place in a stress balance that only slightly or briefly exceeds the load limit.

Here, in turn, appropriate tools have their authority to avoid overloading and to give the autistic person security. For the reasons mentioned above, for example, at school retreats are important that autistic people can visit when needed.

2.6   Dissociative development

A dissociative development or personality structure is what, although unfortunately not uncommon in autistics, cognitive and physical development (age) fit together, but the socio-emotional development at an earlier stage, e.g. due to traumatization, has stopped [Schmidt, B.J .; Ganz, A. (2016)].
The further learning processes in the course of adulthood regarding social interaction did not take place subsequently.
You are then dealing with people who behave intellectually like a (young) adult, but react socio-emotionally like a (defiant) child and sometimes show challenging behavior.
One of the main drawbacks of the previous purely phenomenological-descriptive "understanding" of autism is that the dissociative personality structure was and is equated with autism. As much as one has sought to promote autistic cognitive development, so much has been overlooked for the importance of socio-emotional development and potential risks and obstacles.

Interventions
Again, as with challenging behavior in response to

violence and abuse, prevention is the best intervention. There is a need to change the focus away from cognitive development, which is often unaffected in autistics, toward attention to socio-emotional development. Particular attention should be paid to the "hurdles" of development, for example through changes in caregivers and the social environment, be it through development or external factors such as kindergarten and schooling [Ganz, A .; Schmidt, B.J. (2016)].

If there is already a dissociative personality structure, both therapeutic post-maturation and "social competency training" are recommended [Schmidt, B.J .; Ganz, A. (2016)].

VII.   REVIEW

Finally, let's review the quoted list of challenging behavior under the new perspectives.
"Running away" is usually just running to reduce tension and stress.

Beating, scratching, biting, are auto-aggressive behaviors, especially in children of the "flight" type. These behaviors are also used to reduce anxiety and stress. It is necessary to distinguish the acute action to prevent self-endangerment and a long-term pedagogical-psychological intervention.

social disinterest,
do not speak,
Withdrawal through self-stimulation,
These behaviors often show autistic children of the "flight" type who have withdrawn from a perceived as threatening and incomprehensible world. The consequence of the withdrawal of social interaction is then the disruption of further socio-emotional development.

Disturbance of the day / night rhythm

The day / night rhythm, as part of the development of homeostasis, also depends on a successful orientation towards the social environment.

Threatening, spitting, biting, scratching, hitting.

These behaviors can be found especially in the "fight" children and can be part of a normal as well as disturbed development.

Stereotypical handling of objects.

This creates its own world, which is perceived as safe, and displaces the social world, which is perceived as unsafe and threatening.

make sounds

Can be self-stimulation with the goal of stress reduction, but also the creation of a separate acoustic world against the perceived as incomprehensible outer world.

Rigid insistence on routine.

Is not only found in autistic people, but also in "normal" groups, and serves to avoid anxiety.

Enter into foreign areas, keep no distance, etc.

Is often an expression of the strong exploration urge of

"fight" children and can then be used as a way to build social interaction.

• which are experienced as psychologically conditioned - anxiety, depression, hyperactivity, autism or psychosis, but also self- and auto-aggression, etc.
- compulsive handling of objects

Autism has no place in this list because autism is not a (mental) disease but a vulnerability. On the contrary, it is important to note that even autistic people can develop mental illnesses, indeed the risk is even particularly high. In addition, this list also lacks the dissociative personality structure frequently found in autistics.

[The bold italicized text parts come from: ways to participate - Wege zur Teilhabe – Herausforderndes Verhalten von Menschen mit Behinderungen.

Handreichung des Lebenshilfe-Landesverbandes Bayern 2017]

BIBLIOGRAPHY

Dykema, Ravi (2006):
"Don't talk to me now, I'm scanning for danger"
How your nervous system sabotages your ability to relate
An interview with Stephen Porges about his polyvagal theory.
NEXUS March/April 2006

Menzies Lyth, Isabel (1960): Social Systems as a Defense
Against Anxiety. An Empirical Study of the Nursing Service of a
General Hospital.
In: Human Relations (13), S. 95–121.

Schmidt, Bernhard J. (2015/1): Autistic and Society. An angry Change
of Perspective. Vol. I: Understanding Autism. Norderstedt: Books on
Demand.

Schmidt, Bernhard J. (2015/2): Autistic and Society. An angry Change
of Perspective. Vol. II: Support for Autistic? Norderstedt: Books on
Demand.

Schmidt, Bernhard J. (2016): Plaintext compact. The Asperger
Syndrome – Between Bullying and Inclusion. Norderstedt: Books on
Demand.

Schmidt, Bernhard J.; Ganz, Andreas (2016): Plaintext compact: The
Asperger Syndrome - not only for Psychotherapists. Norderstedt:
Books on Demand.

Schmidt, Bernhard J.; Döhler, Christiane and Deniz (2018): Autism –
Sexuality – Relationships. Norderstedt: Books on Demand.

Schmidt, Bernhard J. (2019/1): Autism and the Refrigerator Mother Myth. A Rehabilitation of Bruno Bettelheim. Norderstedt: Books on Demand.

Schmidt, Bernhard J. (2019/2): Plaintext compact. The Asperger Syndrome – for Parents. Norderstedt: Books on Demand.

Schmidt, Bernhard J. (2019/3): Plaintext compact. The Asperger Syndrome – for Teachers. Norderstedt: Books on Demand.

Schmidt, Bernhard J. (2019/4): Plaintext compact. The Asperger Syndrome – for School Assistants. Norderstedt: Books on Demand.

Schmidt, Bernhard J. (2019/5): Plaintext compact. The Asperger Syndrome – for Physicians. Norderstedt: Books on Demand.

Schmidt, Bernhard J. (2019/6): Practice compact. Autism and Dog. Norderstedt: Books on Demand.

Smith, Peter B.; Bond, Michael Harris (1998):
Social psychology across cultures. 2. Aufl. Harlow [u.a.], Harlow [u.a.]: Prentice Hall Europe.

Turner, John C. (2005): Explaining the nature of power: a three-process theory. In: Eur. J. Soc. Psychol. 35 (1), S. 1–22. DOI: 10.1002/ejsp.244.